Apple Cider Vinegar, Coconut Oil & Almond Oil Miracle

Health and Beauty Secrets You Wish You Knew

Disclaimer

How This eBook Will Change Your Life

Since time immemorial, apple cider vinegar, coconut oil and almond oil have been used not only in cooking, but also in medicines and for other home care purposes. The beneficial properties of these three liquids is so extensive that they have been called miracle cures for many health related issues. All three can be ingested and help with various body functioning and in the cure of multiple diseases.

But that is not the only reason for their popularity. Apple cider vinegar, coconut oil and almond oil also possess huge advantages for the skin and hair. They are the main ingredients for most beauty products because of their ability to slow down the ageing process without any side effects. Why waste hundreds of dollars when you can use them directly? How can you use them and for what purposes? This is exactly what *Health Benefits of Apple Cider Vinegar, Coconut Oil & Almond Oil* will explain to you. This eBook will tell you:

1. The health benefits of apple cider vinegar, coconut oil and almond oil

2. How these liquids should be used in everyday life

3. Which is the best kind of vinegar or oil to use

4. How to improve your skin and hair by the use of these liquids

5. Some simple tips and tricks to help you become fit and gorgeous

When you are done reading this book, you will be equipped with all the information required to become healthy and look beautiful by the use of these wondrous liquids. So instead of just talking about how you can do it, let us explore all the ways you can put your plan into action!

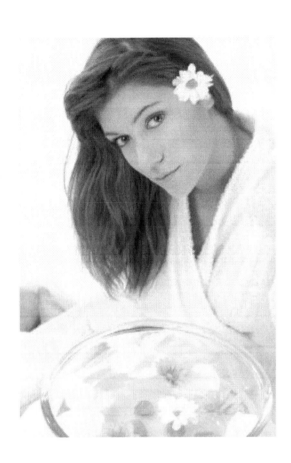

Contents

Introduction

Apple cider vinegar has been in use for a variety of ways since the time of its discovery. It isn't just great for health; it has also been used to clean utensils, get rid of weeds, manufacture pickles, clean armor and of course for cooking. Cider vinegar is used as a toner for skin, as a well as conditioner for oily hair. Recent studies show that there is significant data to prove that the vinegar helps in fighting many diseases such as diabetes, obesity and indigestion. But these are only few of the things that cider vinegar is good for. Suffice it to say, apple cider vinegar hasn't been called the miracle vinegar for no reason.

Just like apple cider vinegar, coconut oil has such benefits that if you make it a part of your regular diet and personal hygiene routine, you will notice a visible difference in your overall fitness and wellbeing. From quickening the process of new tissue development for skin to treating itchy, flaky scalp and working to fight against medical problems like Alzheimer's disease, heart issues, Crohn's disease, thyroid conditions, irritable bowel syndrome and lowering cholesterol, coconut oil can work wonders for literally everyone.

Use of almond oil is likewise just as advantageous as the above mentioned liquids. It helps in the nourishment of skin and hair. Be it hair fall or split ends, lackluster hair or dry and damaged hair, acne prone skin or eczema, dark circles under the eyes or signs of ageing, almond oil is great for all kinds of skin and hair repair.

Entranced? Want to find out more about these miracles of nature? Read on to find out everything

you need to know.

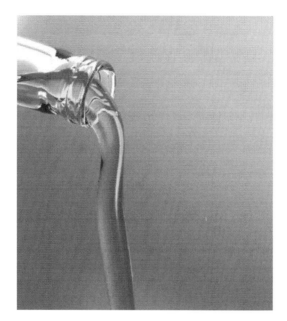

Chapter 1: All You Need to Know about Apple Cider Vinegar

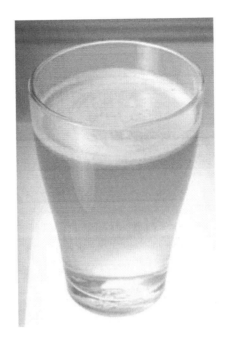

Apple cider vinegar has been in use since at least 10,000 years ago. It is believed that Hippocrates used it as a health tonic. Even the Babylonians used it as a preservative. Chinese and Egyptian histories likewise show the use of vinegar not only in food but in health care as well. Roman military and Japanese samurai used cider vinegar in their drinks, as energy tonics and for antiseptic healing of wounds. American soldiers and sailors, who went sailing with Columbus, also used it as a cure for scurvy, indigestion and pneumonia.

But common man wasn't the only one who benefited from the vinegar. King Louis XIII of France ordered barrels of cider vinegar so that his army could use it to cool down the canons. All this history proves the fact that apple cider vinegar has been in use for centuries because of its multitude of advantages. Below is information on how apple cider vinegar is manufactured.

Some Basic Information

Commercial Manufacturing

It was in 1394 that apple cider vinegar was first commercially manufactured. French vintners came up with the idea of using oak barrels as fermentation vessels. They called this method the Orleans method. The production of apple cider vinegar requires specific ingredients, unlike other forms of vinegars. Main ingredients for the fermentation process are pulverized apples, acetic acid, some minerals and amino acids.

From then on cider vinegar is easily available in the market and can be purchased from any grocery or general store.

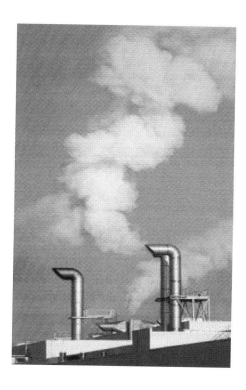

Popularity

Even though apple cider vinegar had been in use since 400 BC, it gained popularity after the publication of Dr. D.C. Jarvis' book "Folk Medicine: A Vermont Doctor's Guide to Good Health" in 1958. In the book, Dr. Jarvis explained how cider vinegar could be used for many purposes including general wellbeing. He claimed that by mixing cider vinegar and honey (a concoction he called honegar), healing prowess of the vinegar multiplied. He also wrote that it was an excellent remedy for bacteria in the digestive tract.

Health Benefits

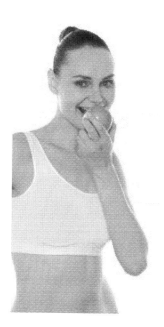

There are dozens of apple cider vinegar health benefits. Some of them are mentioned below. It is recommended that before ingesting the liquid or applying it externally, be sure to consult your medical health practitioner.

Control Blood Cholesterol and Blood Sugars

Is your doctor giving you grief over high cholesterol and blood sugar? Research shows that apple cider vinegar helps in improving the lipid profile and insulin sensitivity. All you have to do is combine 1 teaspoon of vinegar in 1 glass of water and drink it 3 times a day.

Weight Loss

Many studies give evidence for the fact that apple cider vinegar helps in the process of weight loss. What it does is speed up your metabolic rate, which in turn helps in creating a quick digestive system. All you would need to do is mix 2 teaspoons of vinegar in 1 glass of water and drink the solution throughout the day.

Stomach Problems

Are you prone to tummy issues? Well, apple cider vinegar is the perfect cure. Be it diarrhea or intestinal spasms, cider vinegar can help with all. All you have to do is mix one teaspoon of apple cider with 2 spoons of water and drink it. It also helps to relieve acid reflux before it even starts. Just take a spoonful with water before eating.

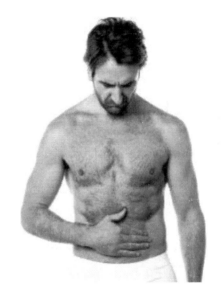

Clear Sinus

Have you been going through bad flu symptoms? Can't breathe properly because of a stuffy nose? Just take one glass of water and mix 1 teaspoon of cider vinegar in it. Gulp down and feel the sinuses clear!

Sore Throat

Is a sore threat threatening to ruin your weekend? Take out the bottle of apple cider vinegar from your kitchen cupboard and mix ¼ cup of it with ¼ cup of water. Start gargling away!

Yeast Infections and Fungi

Have you developed a yeast infection? You don't need to buy expensive creams and lotions, just take out the apple cider vinegar from the cupboard. Fill up your bathtub with warm water and add 1 ½ cups of cider vinegar in it. Soak for about 20 minutes for 3 days and see results.

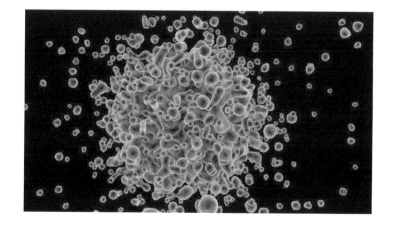

Teeth Cleaner

Apple cider vinegar can be a great tool for cleaning your teeth. All you need to do is take some in a cup and rub it directly on your teeth. Leave it on for 30 seconds and rinse your mouth thoroughly. The acid helps in killing off bacteria and removing stains from the teeth.

Energy Booster

Cider vinegar helps in maintaining the equilibrium of your body. Research suggests that it helps in reducing the alkalinity of the body and thus the pH of your body becomes regular. This in turn helps increase energy and makes you more active. If you ingest 1 tsp in the morning, you will see visible differences.

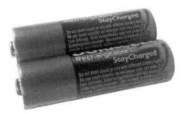

Hiccups

Since hiccups are a reason of indigestion, the use of apple cider vinegar is the ideal solution.

Heartburn

If you have been a lifelong patient of acid reflux and heartburn, then forget the multitude of antacids you have been consuming and concentrate on cider vinegar instead. What the vinegar does is control the amount of acid rolling around in your stomach by neutralizing its effects. As soon as you feel the heartburn, ingest 1 teaspoon of cider vinegar and drink a glass full of water immediately afterwards.

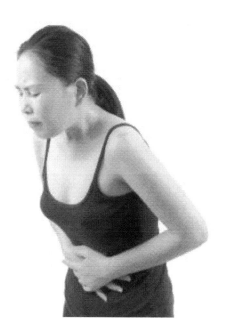

Lymphatic System

Apple cider vinegar helps clear your sinus because it aids in the breakdown of mucous throughout the body. This results in the clearing of lymph nodes. So if you are prone to allergies, cider vinegar can become your best friend! It also keeps diseases like sore throats, flu, sinus infection and

headaches at bay.

Swelling

If you have been experiencing swelling in your feet or hands due to pregnancy or because of

arthritis, try rubbing apple cider vinegar on the swelled body part. You will notice a visible

difference in a few days.

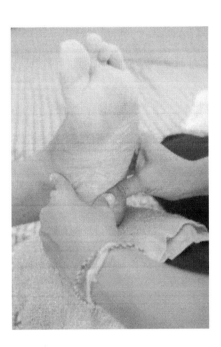

Candida

Have you been suffering from Candida? If yes, then do not stress anymore. You don't have a cause

for fear because apple cider vinegar is here to save the day! Candida is the reason why many people complain of having poor memory, yeast infections, sugar cravings and fatigue. Since cider vinegar is a rich source of natural enzymes, it helps in controlling the disease.

Night Leg Cramps

Ever woke up from a deep, peaceful sleep to an extremely painful leg cramp? It can be excruciating! The best solution is to drink water diluted with apple cider vinegar twice a day. What this does is dissolve acid crystals in your blood, as well as restores the body's supply of potassium, calcium and many other essential minerals. With time you will not suffer from the painful problem.

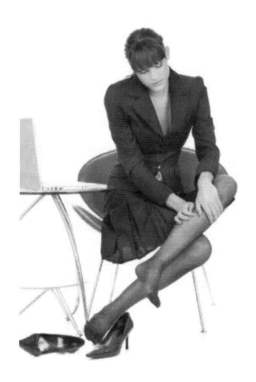

Halitosis

Had halitosis for years? Also known as bad breath, people who have acidic conditions mostly suffer from it. There is a very simple solution for it. Mix 1 cup of water with ½ tablespoon of apple cider vinegar and gargle with this mixture for 10 seconds each time you brush your teeth. Continue till you use up all the solution. Make sure you gargle with plain water afterwards.

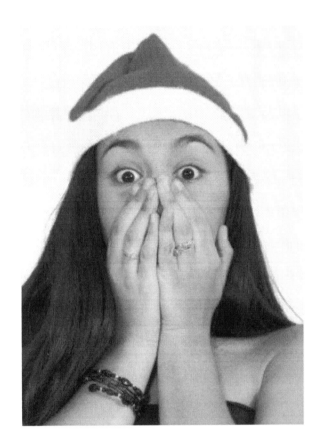

Varicose Veins

Varicose veins don't only look bad they also hurt a lot. Experts suggest that apple cider vinegar can be an excellent remedy for this painful problem. Combine equal parts cider vinegar and your regular lotion and apply to your varicose veins every day, day and night. Make sure you do this in a circular motion. You will see visible results in a month and in due time the issue can completely

disappear.

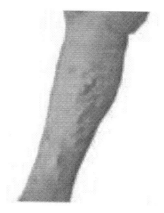

Apple Cider for Skin

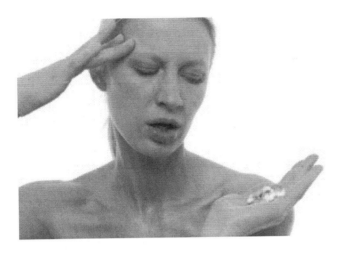

Apple cider vinegar can be the perfect solution to most of your skin problems. Here are some of its uses to enhance your beauty.

Detoxification

Thinking of visiting the spa for a facial and full body detox? There is absolutely no need if you have apple cider vinegar lying at home. All you need to do is fill your tub with warm water, your choice of liquid soap and add 1 ½ cups of vinegar to it. Soak for at least 20-30 minutes and feel your body become soft and supple.

For a face mask you would need 2 tablespoon apple cider vinegar, 2 tablespoon bentonite clay and 1 tablespoon honey. Mix well and apply to face, leaving for 10-15 minutes. Wash off with warm water.

Toner

Since apple cider vinegar contains acetic acid, it also works well as a toner. What makes it the best is its antibacterial properties.

Acne and Age Spots

Acne and age spots can be a real pain for women of all ages. Cider vinegar helps in fighting bacteria from accumulating on oily skin, as well as reduces the effects of ageing. Just dab some on the affected area and leave overnight. Wash off in the morning.

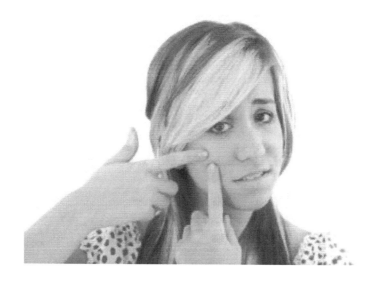

Saves you from Sun Burn

If you want to get rid of that horrendous sun burn, let apple cider vinegar save your day! Just dip some cotton balls in vinegar and apply to affected places. It will ease the sting and help heal the peeling skin faster.

Vinegar for Feet

Are the effects of high heels taking their toll on your feet? Prepare an invigorating foot soak by mixing 1 part vinegar and 1 part warm water and soaking your feet for 30 minutes. Wash off with cool water afterwards. This is also a great relief provider for pregnant ladies.

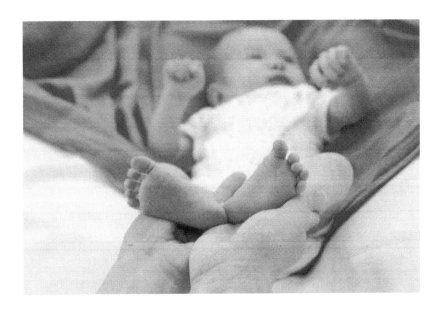

Mosquito bites, Cuts or Abrasions

Have mosquito bites that refuse to disappear? Keep getting cuts and abrasions on your hands and feet? Is your skin sore and irritated? Apple cider vinegar is a cure for all these problems. Simply combine equal parts of water and cider vinegar and apply to the irritated skin. You will notice that with continued use, the irritation and redness disappears.

For Warts

If you think that wart removal is very expensive, try opting for apple cider vinegar instead. Not only is it extremely cheap, it is also very effective. All you need to do is dip a cotton ball in apple cider vinegar until it soaks through and then place it on the wart. Cover it with a bandage and leave overnight. Do this for a week and you will notice results.

Inexpensive Aftershave!

Do you want to get rid of expensive aftershaves? Apple cider vinegar is the perfect solution. Simply combine some with equal amounts of water in a spray bottle and give your face a sprinkle after shaving!

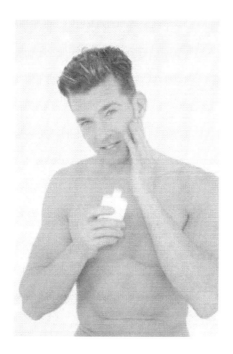

Skin Whitening

Did you know that cider vinegar is used as a natural skin whitener too? Hard to believe? Try it!

All you need to do is mix equal parts of water and vinegar and apply it to your face twice daily.

After 10 days you will see a visible difference and can continue until you achieve desired results.

Do not use cider vinegar directly on your skin. Always dilute with water first.

Soft, Smooth Skin

If you want to have skin like silk then add vinegar to your lotion. Simply combine equal amounts

of apple cider vinegar and your lotion, mix well and use daily. This will not only soften your skin,

it will also help in giving you a clear, beautiful complexion.

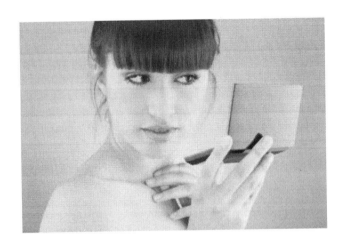

Apple Cider for Hair

Skin isn't the only part of your body that benefits from the external use of apple cider vinegar. Here are some ways you can make your hair shinier, softer and healthier with cider vinegar.

Soft and Shiny Hair

Apple cider vinegar works wonders as a conditioner. Unlike commercial chemical conditioners, there is absolutely no chance of damage either. Once you have shampooed your hair, rinse with a mixture of cider vinegar and water. To make the rinse, combine ½ cup of vinegar with 4 cups of water. Pour this mixture over hair, leave in for 2 minutes and then rinse with cold water. You will see results then and there.

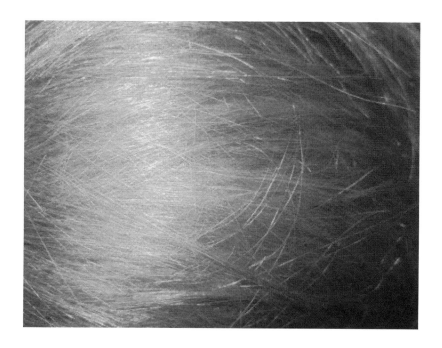

Improve Hair Growth

Apple cider vinegar is said to improve hair growth. You can use it after washing your hair with baking soda and see a difference within 1 month. Make sure you don't use vinegar more than 2 times a week.

Get Tangle Free

Got hair that tangles too easily? You can combine 1 tablespoon of vinegar with 1 glass of water and put it in a spray bottle. Spray lightly on hair, leave for 2 minutes and then comb.

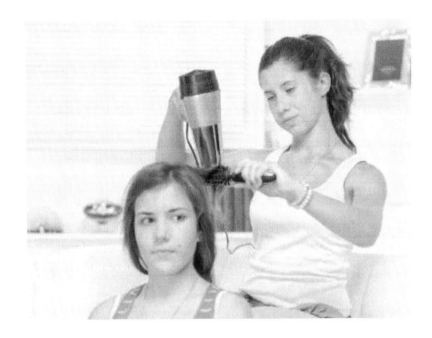

Itchy Scalp

Only people who are scratching their heads all the time can understand the pain of an itchy and dry scalp. If you too have been going through the same problem, try using apple cider vinegar. Since it has antibacterial and antifungal properties, it can work well for dry scalp, giving it the nutrients required for healing.

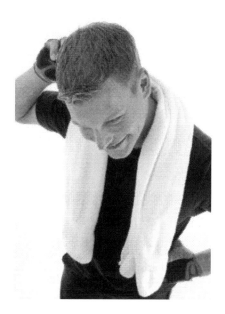

Hair Cleanser

Apple cider vinegar is considered to be one of the most effective hair cleansers. It gets rid of all the residue and helps clean your hair from the inside out. Just combine cider vinegar with baking soda and wash it like washing with shampoo. Make sure you rinse thoroughly.

Frizz Treatment

If you have hair that frizzes easily in winters or otherwise, apple cider vinegar can be great for you. Whether you have dry or oily hair, cider vinegar can work wonders for all conditions.

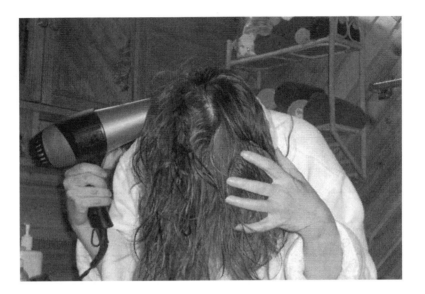

Some Easy to Use Tips and Tricks

These easy recipes and tricks are the perfect way to get a beautiful you, as well as a great house!

You will find everything easily in the market and won't have to spend more than $5!

Lasting Nail Color

Do you want your nail color to last longer than a few hours? Well then, apple cider can do the trick. Before applying the nail color, take half a cup of warm water with 2 teaspoons of cider vinegar in it. Dip your finger nails in for 2 minutes and then dry off. Apply nail color and see it last for days!

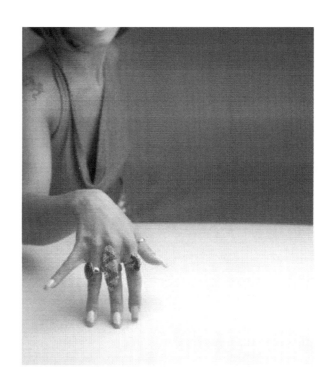

Face Mask

Apple cider vinegar can be great as a face mask. It has anti-ageing and antiseptic properties so it can keep your facial skin young, healthy and free from germs.

Take 2 tablespoons of honey and mix it with 1 tablespoon of cider vinegar. Then apply to face and let sit for about 20 minutes. Wash off with warm water and let dry naturally.

Do this twice to thrice a week to see best results. Make sure you make it a part of your routine facial care treatment.

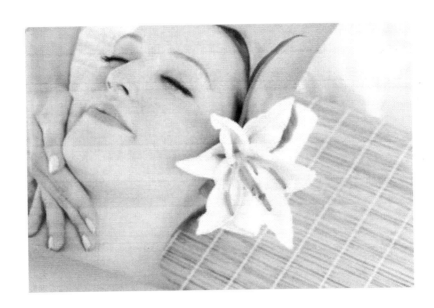

Herbal Hair Conditioner

No conditioner can work as well as cider vinegar. To make it even more effective and sweet smelling, take 1 part apple cider vinegar, 2 parts water and some chopped herbs of your choice.

All you will need to do is bring the herbs to a boil in water, let cool, add cider vinegar and strain.

Then wash your hair after taking a bath with this mixture. Let dry naturally and feel blessed with amazing hair!

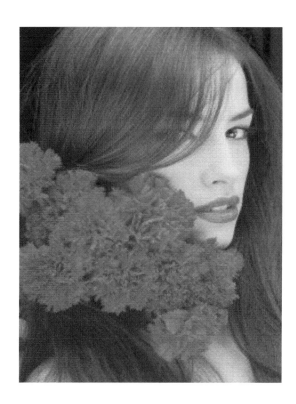

Odorless Fridge

Did you know that vinegar is the best remedy for a smelly refrigerator? White vinegar works too but apple cider vinegar not only reduces the smell but it also helps in killing off bacteria and other germs.

All you have to do is take some apple cider vinegar in a small bowl and put it in a lower shelf of your refrigerator. What the vinegar will do is absorb all the bad smell and leave your fridge odor less.

Keep in mind though that it would work more effectively if you change the vinegar after every month or so.

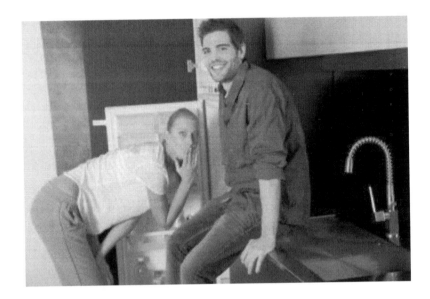

Perfect Toner

Since apple cider vinegar is made up of acid, it is a great toner. It firms up the skin and leaves it looking young and fresh without the effect of any harsh chemicals. Although you can directly apply it to the face as a toner, you can also make it more exotic by using the following recipe.

Take 1 part apple cider vinegar, 2 parts water, 2 drops of almond oil and 2 drops of chamomile essential oil. Mix together and dip a cotton ball in it. Use on a clean face and leave to dry. You can also store it in a spray bottle and sprinkle some on the face after cleansing. It will immediately freshen up your face!

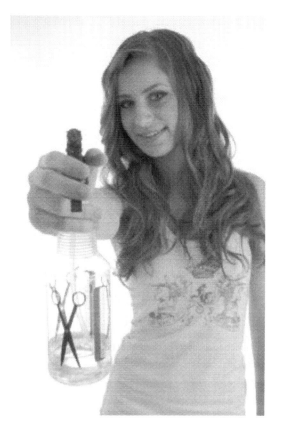

Insect Repellent

Tired of getting insect bites all the time and don't know how to get rid of the bite marks and keep

the insects away? Apple cider can be your savior. Simply mix some in almond oil and apply to

your body whenever you go out camping! It will not only protect you from insect bites, it will also

get rid of all the bite marks!

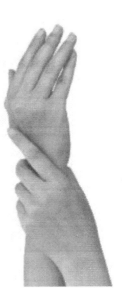

Which Type of Apple Cider to Use

Apple cider vinegar is available in three forms, raw, refined and in the form of solidified pills or capsules. Most experts recommend that you avoid the use of capsules as they contain added preservatives.

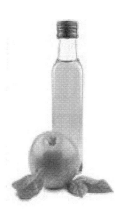

For Internal Use

When you use apple cider vinegar in your cooking or as preservative for pickles, you can use the one easily available in the market. Buying the raw, natural cider vinegar insures that you are at no risk of being harmed by added preservatives.

You can distinguish this one from others by looking at the bottle. If there are residues lying at the bottom, then that means cider is in its raw, organic form.

If you use vinegar for ingestion with water, be 100% sure that the vinegar is in its unadulterated form.

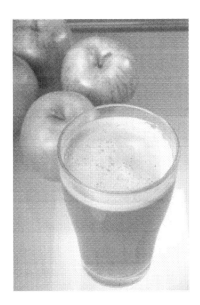

For External Use

If you are using apple cider vinegar for your hair and skin, then too it would be best to use the vinegar in its raw form. But if the usage is for cleaning, washing or other purposes, then you can use whichever type of vinegar is easily available.

Always keep in mind that apple cider vinegar is very strong, so don't use more than the suggested amount.

Chapter 2: All You Need to Know about Coconut Oil

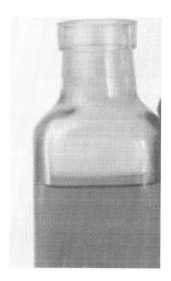

Coconut is one of the most happily devoured fruits. It has many health benefits but the oil extracted from coconut is what is truly its most essential part. Coconut oil is scientifically proven to be a cure for various diseases and ailments. Coconut itself and its oil have been in use since the time man first discovered its tree. From then on it has been used to treat medical conditions, skin problems, hair issues and much, much more.

There came a time in history when coconut oil was shunned, due to the misconception that it was leading to rising coronary diseases. But hundreds of studies have concluded the fact that unlike other saturated fats, coconut oil is easily digested and improves the absorption of other nutrients. In other words, coconut oil is the safest oil on earth!

Some Basic Information

The reason why coconut oil has been hailed as this miraculous liquid is that even though it comes from a family of saturated oils, it still does not cause any weight gain, high blood cholesterol or high blood sugar. Instead coconut oil helps in fighting off all of these problems. The best part about coconut and its oil is that it can even be used by those who are technically on a diet. Since it tastes delicious in all its forms, whether it be coconut meat, milk, water, oil, flour or creamed. Coconut is the best alternative for dairy milk and cream, white flour, vegetable oil, and sweeteners. What's more, it gives some amazing health benefits.

Haven't adopted coconut in your daily life yet? Read on to find out all the health, skin and hair benefits of using coconut oil in your daily diet.

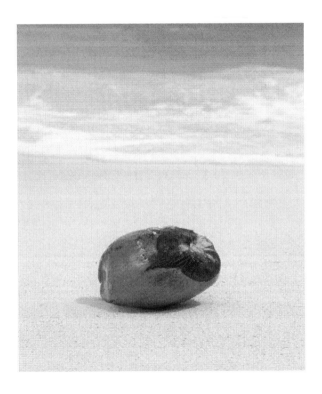

When it comes to health benefits of coconut oil, there are multiple. Some of them have been explained below.

Diabetes Type II

What the oil does is help manage blood sugars and improve insulin secretion. But there's more. Coconut oil also helps in utilizing blood glucose quickly and efficiently.

Helps with Weight Loss

Coconut oil is said to work well for weight loss. Since there are short and medium-chain fatty acids in the oil, they remain easy to digest and do not get stored in the body in the form of fat deposits. They also increase the rate of metabolic activity, which as you must have noticed that people living in the tropics are almost never fat!

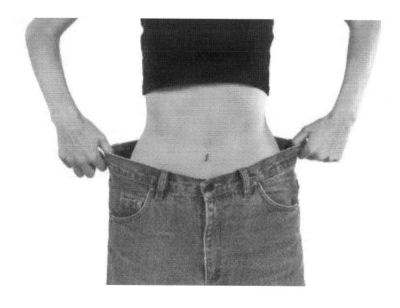

Reduces Seizures

Coconut oil is also said to be beneficial for people who suffer from epilepsy because it helps in reducing seizures. Research suggests that if introduced in the diet of children who have epilepsy, the seizures could be reduced significantly.

Helps Fight Cancer and HIV

Coconut oil helps in improving immunity to viruses and bacteria, which means that it plays a significant role in keeping you safe from HIV, as well as cancer.

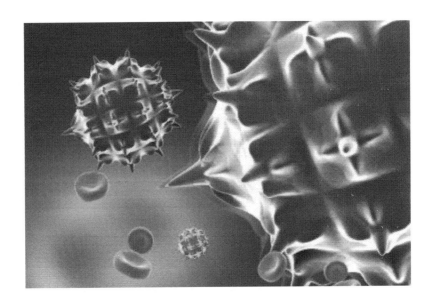

Skin Problems

Research suggests that coconut oil is not just great for weight loss, but also for the health of your skin. It fights off diseases like acne, psoriasis, rosacea, keratosis, and eczema. It is also said to reduce fungal infection. You can either ingest it or apply it directly to the place of infection. Daily application will show wonderful results within no time.

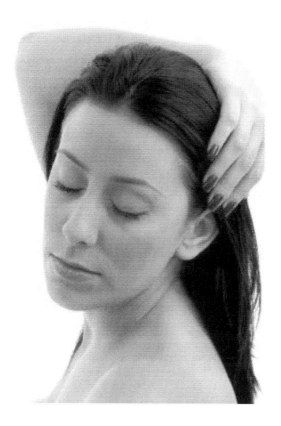

Hypothyroidism

Since coconut oil is effective in boosting metabolism and raising body temperature, it is beneficial in keeping the thyroid and its enzyme secretion regular. This is the reason it can work very well for people who are suffering from hypothyroidism.

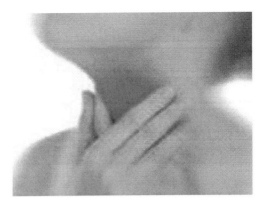

Energy Boost

Feel too tired and fatigued on a day to day basis? Why not try using something natural instead of going for drugs? Coconut oil can be the easiest way of getting energy without consuming any kind of drugs. The best thing though is that it increases endurance, letting you feel fresh and active throughout the day. This is the reason why so many athletes and fitness trainers use this as a type of energy tonic.

Reduced Risk of Heart Ailments

Coconut oil is proposed to reduce the LDL cholesterol and increases HDL which means that it keeps the cholesterol as well as blood pressure under control. This means that the risks of having a heart problem are drastically reduced. Some studies suggest that coconut oil also helps in strengthening the heart muscles allowing the heart to work even better. This is one of the major reasons why it is suggested that you use it in cooking.

Kills off Bacteria and Viruses

Coconut oil contains Lauric Acid and monolaurin that help in the killing off of many pathogens that can be harmful, like bacteria, viruses and many fungi. This helps in making your immune system stronger, giving you more power to fight off infectious diseases.

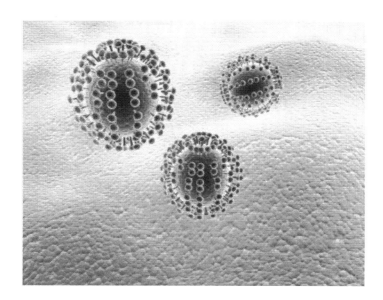

Ear Infection

Has your child, sister, father, spouse been complaining of earaches for a while now? Well it must be an infection then. Just pour a few drops of coconut 2 times a day into the affected ear and see the infection vanish within no time at all!

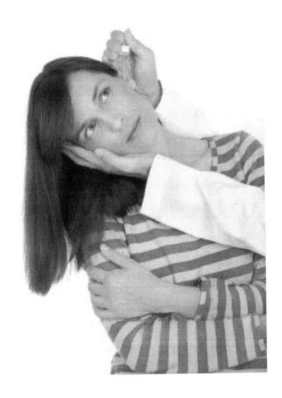

Sleep Problems

Having difficulty going to sleep because of one reason or the other? Why not start ingesting coconut oil almost daily? Studies show that people who use coconut oil in their daily diet find it a lot easier to sleep than others.

Great for Bones

Many studies prove that coconut oil helps in greater absorption of calcium and magnesium which means that your bones are automatically saved from arthritis or any other bone condition!

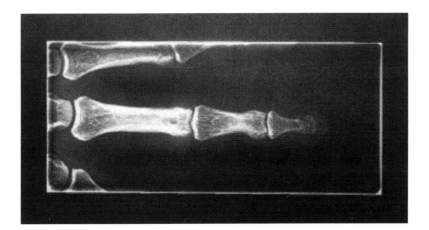

For a Healthier You!

Coconut oil isn't called a miracle cure for nothing! It has many benefits that keep both the mind

and body healthy. Whether you use it in your cooking, take it directly or apply it to the skin or

hair, coconut oil can be beneficial in all its uses. Another great thing about this oil is that it

generates a healthy you and improves the quality of life!

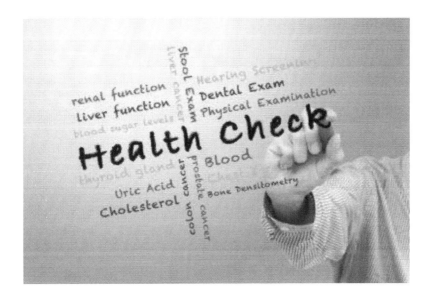

Prevents and Reverses Alzheimer's

Recent studies show that coconut oil can be great for all those who are at risk of developing Alzheimer's disease. The interesting thing though is that it not only helps in preventing the degenerative disease, but it also helps in reversing the condition. Even though more research is required to be absolutely sure about this; the studies that have been conducted show positive results. This could be a real breakthrough as yet there is still no cure for Alzheimer's.

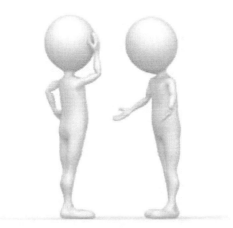

Coconut Oil for Pets

Did you know that coconut oil is not just great for human use but animals too? It is generally accepted that coconut oil is good for pets because it helps improve their immune system, digestion and bone health. It can also be used on any cuts or abrasions your pets receive.

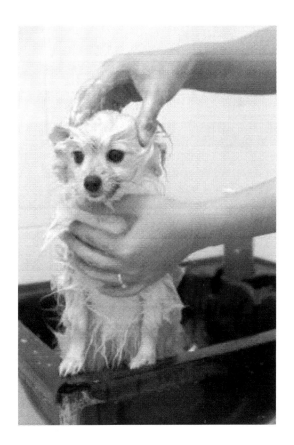

Coconut Oil for Skin

Many people, research analysts and experts included, hail coconut oil as the miracle product for skin. Be it dry or oily, acne prone or T-zone mix, coconut oil can be great for all kinds of skin types. Below are some ways you can use coconut oil for your skin.

Tablespoon of Coconut a Day

If you aren't already taking it, then now is the right time to start. Have you heard of the famous Australian model Miranda Kerr? She is known for her glowing, spotless skin and glossy hair. She swears by the power of coconut oil. Ms. Kerr has emphasized many times that the reason for her gorgeous hair and skin is the ingestion of 4 tablespoons of coconut oil daily.

It is recommended to men and women alike that they should include coconut oil in their regular diets.

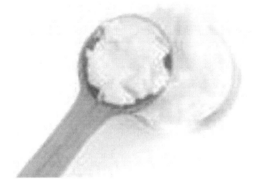

Delays Ageing

Coconut oil is the perfect remedy for wrinkles and sagging skin. You can massage it on your face as well as the rest of your body and see visible results within 2 months of use. What it does is slow down the process of ageing.

Perfect Moisturizer

No more do you need to buy expensive products to hydrate your skin. Just pour a small amount of coconut oil in your palm and rub it on your face. Because coconut oil is lightweight, it gets absorbed in the skin easily, leaving you with a soft and glowing look.

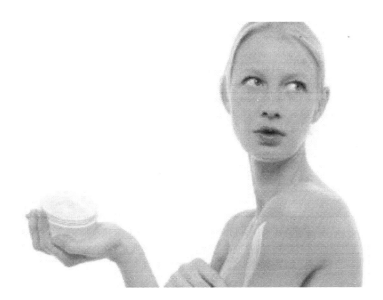

For Problematic Skin

Coconut oil is also believed to be great for skin conditions like acne, acne scars, eczema, dermatitis, psoriasis and many other infections. This is the reason why it is used in so many skin care products.

Reduces Fine Lines

Did you know that coconut oil is also great for treating fine lines and wrinkles? You simply have to take some and gently rub into the areas that you see fine lines in. Better to do this at night as that would mean you won't have to keep dabbing the oil off your face, if you have an oily skin complexion.

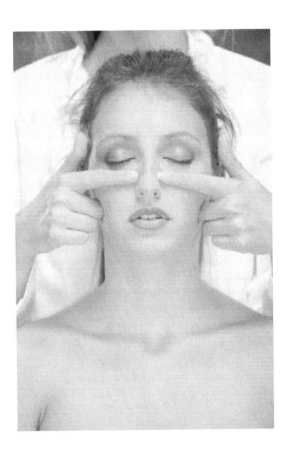

Makeup Remover

Stop wasting money on expensive makeup removers that contain millions of chemicals which are extremely dangerous for you. Instead opt for coconut oil, a natural makeup remover. You will only have to put some on a cotton ball and apply to your face. Do wash your face after removing the makeup and then lightly apply a coat of the oil in place of a night cream. You will wake up to gorgeous, soft skin.

Natural Chap Stick

How can coconut not have something for your lips as well if it does so many things for other body parts? Since the oil is naturally semi solid at room temperature, it can easily be stored in a small bottle and used on your lips whenever you feel they are getting dry! It works better than any commercial chap stick you might have tried before!

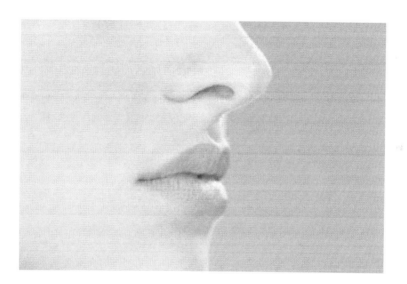

Stretch Marks

Coconut oil should be the best friend of every pregnant lady as it helps in preventing and reducing stretch lines. All you need to do is rub coconut oil all over your body or in the places where you have stretch marks. A small tip is that instead of waiting for the stretch marks to appear, start applying coconut oil in your second trimester. This will greatly reduce the risks of having them develop in the first place.

Cellulite

If you have been suffering from cellulite and nothing seems to work for you, start applying coconut oil today. Keep using it and you will notice that slowly and gradually the condition starts receding.

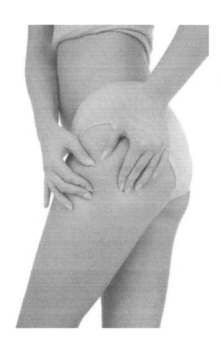

For Sensitive Skin

If you are among those who can apply nothing on their skin because of irritation and redness, try coconut oil. It's so mild it will never harm you in any possible way! All you will need to do is rub it in your skin.

Diaper Cream

Is your baby crying every day because of those huge red rashes? Too worried the chemical creams might be dangerous? Worry no more! Simply use coconut oil in place of the diaper cream and see the rashes disappear within days!

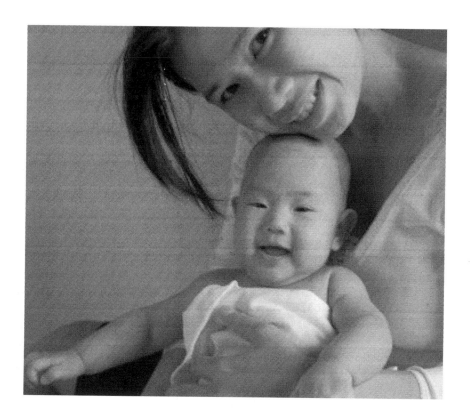

Dry Hands and Feet

Do you suffer from overly dry hands and feet? Well coconut oil is there to rescue you. Simply take some and massage gently on your hands and feet. The best time would be just before you go to bed. Rub your hands and feet with the oil and wear socks and gloves. You will wake up the next day with soft, dewy hands and feet!

Nail Growth

If you have weak nails or are having difficulty in growing them, try applying coconut oil to them every day. Your nails will strengthen, as well as harden, allowing you to grow them as long as you want.

Sun Protection

If you aren't a fan of sunscreen lotions, then use coconut oil instead. The oil acts as a natural protection from the hazardous rays of the sun, and keeps you safe from sun burning.

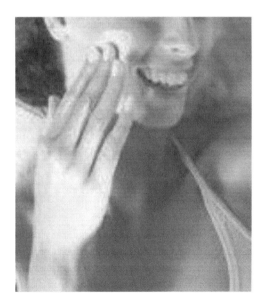

Coconut Oil for Hair

As mentioned before, coconut oil is also great for your hair. Here are some of its uses.

Super Shiny and Soft Hair

Coconut oil is a great hair conditioner. All you need to do is take some coconut oil, warm it up, massage into your scalp and cover with a showering cap. Then leave it for overnight if you can. If you don't have the time, then let the oil penetrate the scalp for half an hour. Wash off and enjoy the feel of your soft, shiny hair.

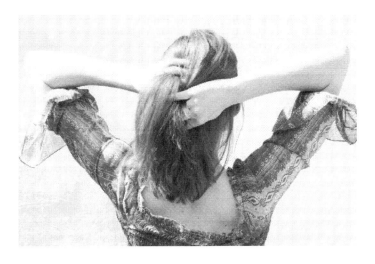

Locks in Moisture

The reason why hair gets dry is because moisture evaporates. With regular use of coconut oil, your hair starts retaining some of the moisture necessary to keep it looking lustrous. It keeps the impurities out and helps make your hair healthy.

For Hair Growth

Coconut oil is rich in Vitamin E, K and Iron which not only reduce dandruff; it also nourishes the hair allowing them to grow longer and stronger. Just make sure you massage the oil in your scalp twice a week.

Get Rid of the Static

Hate the feeling when your hair seems to be standing on end in Winter? This is caused due to dryness and static. Just take some coconut oil in your hand and rub it on your hair. But only take a small amount or your hair will feel oily.

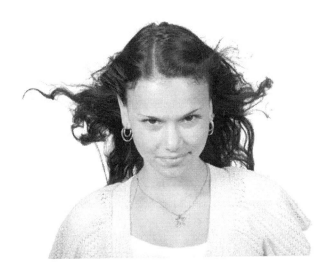

Split Ends

If your hair is getting damaged because of all the dust, air and chemical usage, try massaging some coconut oil in it. It not only reverses all kinds of damage, it also helps in reducing split ends.

Lusterless Hair Solution

Have you been recently told that your hair looks like they had died? Instead of getting offended, look for reasons and solutions. Again coconut oil can save your hair from dying completely. Just warm some up and apply to hair. Leave for an hour or two and then wash off. You will feel as if a new life has been blessed to your hair!

Saves Your from Scalp Conditions

Coconut oil is not only great for the hair; it is also wonderful for your scalp and hair follicles. If you have developed eczema or other scalp conditions, coconut oil can be the remedy for you. Just pour some oil in your hand and rub in your scalp. You will notice a difference within a few weeks!

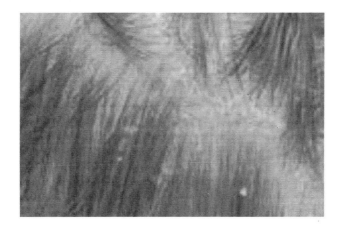

Lice Solution

Did your daughter just catch lice from the girl next door? Want to control the problem before it spreads like a wild fire? Start massaging coconut oil in her hair and the lice will be gone before you know it! You can also mix some apple cider vinegar in it to see better results.

Gets Rid of Dandruff

Coconut oil is a natural remedy for dandruff. Forget those expensive, chemical ridden shampoos and give your itchy scalp a warm coconut oil treatment. You will find results after the third wash!

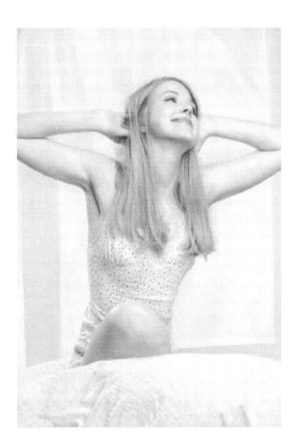

Some Easy to Use Tips and Tricks

Here are a few recipes and tips that would not only be very affordable but will also work a lot better than anything you buy from the market. Keep in mind that you should only use the quantities that are mentioned. If you plan to ingest the oil, then be sure to ask your doctor first.

Coconut Moisturizer

If you have dry skin or normal skin, then this moisturizer is great for you. The best part? You can make it right at home! Just take 2 cups of coconut oil and whip it on high in the mixer. Then when it has softened, add 2 drops of lavender essential oil and 2 drops of tea tree essential oil. Whip until fluffy then store in a jar. Use as needed. It is best used before sleeping and once you have washed your face in the morning.

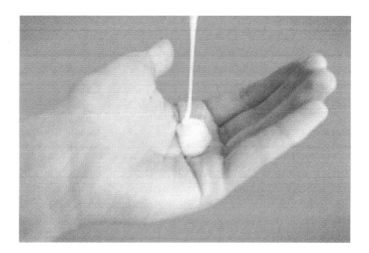

Deodorant

Want to get rid of offending body odor but don't have the money to spend too much money on expensive deodorants? Well why not make your own? Sounds crazy? It most certainly is not. All you need to do is gather some important ingredients and remain happy and odor free forever!

Combine 1/3 cup coconut oil, 1/3 cup arrowroot powder and 2 tbsp baking soda together and mix until it turns to the consistency of deodorant. You can also add 15 drops of your favorite essential oils to give the deodorant your favorite scent. The great thing about this deodorant is that it works wonderfully for sensitive skin too.

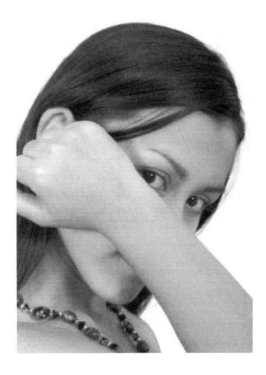

Coconut Lip Balm

Coconut makes for an excellent lip balm if used directly. But if you want to make it more effective and interesting, try this recipe given below.

Take 1 tablespoon coconut oil, 1 tablespoon beeswax and 1 tablespoon olive oil and heat in a glass container. When all the oils are melted and well combined, pour in a small container and let cool. It will solidify and you can use it easily.

If you want the lip balm to have some color, all you need to do is add a pinch of your favorite color when the oils have heated completely and mix well.

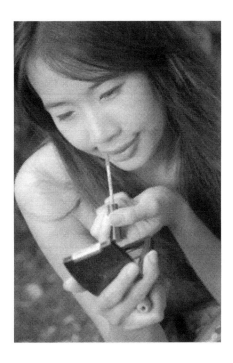

Hair Mask

Tired of your falling, dull and lifeless hair? Try this homemade coconut hair mask and watch your hair transform within no time. Here is how you can make this mask.

Take 1 tablespoon coconut oil, 1 tablespoon raw honey, and warm it up together. Allow to cool and apply to damp hair. Make sure all the hair roots are completely covered. Cover with a shower cap and leave on 40 minutes. Wash off with warm water and shampoo, then let cold water run through your hair. Let dry and see your hair shine!

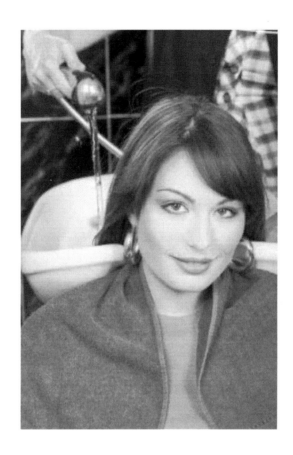

Homemade Brown Eyeliner

Did you know that you can make your very own eye liner with coconut oil? Can there really be anything better? Not only will it be extremely cheap, it will also be totally chemical free. So how can you make it? Here is the simple recipe.

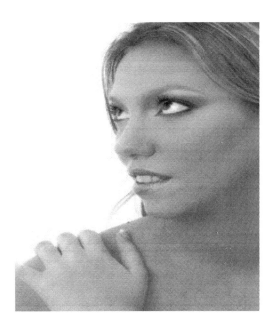

Just take 2 teaspoons of coconut oil, 4 tablespoons of aloe vera gel and ½ teaspoon of cocoa powder. Mix them all up and store in an air tight container. Use with a brush and see amazing results. If you want to make black eyeliner, use 2 capsules of activated charcoal instead of cocoa powder. You can also try other colors to see various results.

Coconut Body Butter

This yummy body butter will literally make you want to eat it, it's that good. Try it and use it after every bath to attain a beautifully soft body!

Simply combine un-melted coconut oil, a few drops of tea tree essential oil and some drops of ylang ylang essential oil and whip on high for 7-8 minutes. Keep in a lidded jar and store at room temperature.

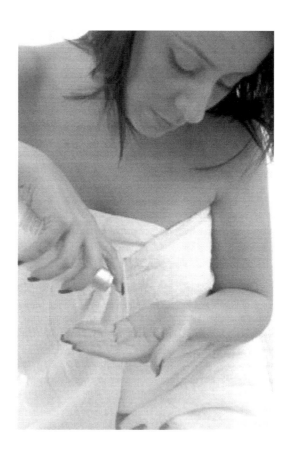

Which Type of Coconut Oil to Use

There are many varieties of coconut oil available in the market. It is essential that you use the right oil in the right place; otherwise the results may not be as great as you expect. Below is a list of different kinds of coconut oil and which one you should use where.

1. **Pure Coconut Oil:** one of the most commonly used and oldest forms of coconut oil, the pure version is great for a variety of purposes. It is extracted from the dried kernel of coconuts, known as copra. The oil is edible.

2. **Virgin Coconut Oil:** By far the tastiest form of coconut oil, it is extracted by the process of fermentation, from fresh coconut meat. It is highly rich in antioxidants and has wonderful microbial properties.

3. **Organic Coconut Oil:** Another widely used variety, organic coconut oil is as harmless as they come. From growth of the coconut tree to the process of oil extraction and storage, there is no chemical involved in the production of this oil. This is the reason why it is used in most personal hygiene and beauty care products.

4. **Refined Coconut Oil:** This type of coconut oil is manufactured chemically and it is best that you avoid its usage for health care. It is the refined, bleached and deodorized form of coconut oil.

5. **Carrier Oil:** Coconut oil is also used as a base oil or carrier oil. This is the reason why it is popular for therapies like Aromatherapy, Chinese medicine, Ayurveda and many other kinds of massages and spa treatments. Because of its anti-bacterial, anti-fungal properties, as well as its stability, it is combined with many other essential oils and stored for years without any fear of the concoction going rancid.

So which oil should you use?

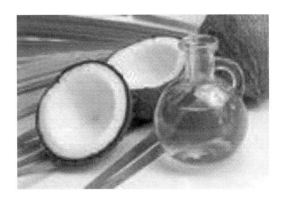

For Internal Use

If you directly want to ingest coconut oil whether for general good health, weight loss or prettier skin, go for virgin oil. This is best because it is free from all kinds of chemicals or preservatives.

For External Use

For external use like applying oil on your hair, skin or for massages, you can use either pure coconut oil or refined coconut oil. They work equally well. Even if you go for organic or virgin, they too would work equally well but they will cost more.

Chapter 3: All You Need to Know about Almond Oil

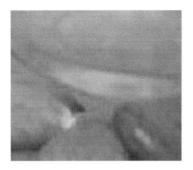

In recent years, almond oil has been gaining a lot of popularity. And there are some very solid

reasons for this. What is interesting to note is that even though almond oil just recently came into

commercial use, it has been around since before the Christian era. Many studies of ancient history

suggest that in 3000 and 2000 B.C. or what is known as the Bronze Age, almond oil was discovered

by man and used for its nut, seeds, as well as oil. The oil has also been mentioned in Greek and

Italian histories, as well as in the Bible. Its properties and use was also mentioned in Greek

mythology and Shakespearean writings.

The most important thing to keep in mind about almond oil is that there are two types available.

One is extracted from the sweet almond tree that is a favorite snack among nut lovers, while the

other is taken from bitter almond tree, which can be poisonous if ingested in large amounts.

Also keep in mind that bitter almond oil is an essential oil and it not safe for use on skin or hair, it

is only used for aroma and flavor. But even then a few drops go a long way, because the oil is very powerful. Even though it does not have any extra property or healing powers, bitter almond oil is loved for its scent.

Another warning before the use of almond oil is that you should be very sure you are not allergic to it. If you are then almond oil is not for you. Be sure to consult your medical health practitioner before using the oil.

It is the sweet almond oil that has multiple health, skin and hair benefits. Below is all the information you would need.

Some Basic Information

You might wonder that if almond oil is so wonderful why is it only now that it has gained popularity? A simple answer is that it was only recently that proper research was conducted on it.

The reason why almond oil is so beneficial is that it is made up of olein, linoleic acid and glucosides. All these give almond oil its rich nutritional value, making it high in proteins, vitamins and minerals. It is considered to be one of the best skin care products on earth!

Since the oil is light, it is easily absorbed by the skin leaving only a sheen or oily coating on your face. But keep in mind that all of this is for sweet almond oil only. If you end up putting bitter almond oil on your skin, you might have a severe reaction.

Health Benefit

There are numerous health benefits of almond oil. Some of them are stated below.

Heart Friendly

Almond oil is a great source of folic acid, potassium and mono-saturated proteins and fats, which make it excellent for heart patients. All you have to do is add 1 teaspoon to your regular cooking oil.

Effective Laxative

If you have a weak digestive system and have stomach troubles, then you can start taking one teaspoon of almond oil before dinner every two days. This will improve your digestion.

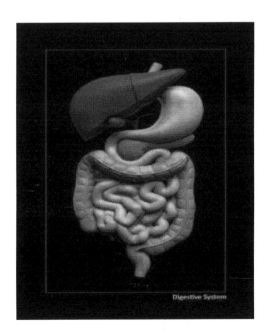

Strong Nervous System and Memory

You must have heard how eating raw almonds can be great for your memory. Well the same is the case with almond oil. But it gets better because almond oil also strengthens your nervous system. Just add two drops in a glass of warm milk and take it at least 3 days a week.

Analgesic Properties

Did you know that almond oil also works as a pain reliever? Not only does it ease pain, it also helps in relaxing of the muscles. All you would need to do is heat up the oil and massage it into the area that feels sore or painful. It is particularly great for neck pain, knee joints, arthritic patients, as well as the elderly. If you have painful heels or tired feet, just give yourself a warm almond oil massage and then soak your feet in warm water infused with almond oil.

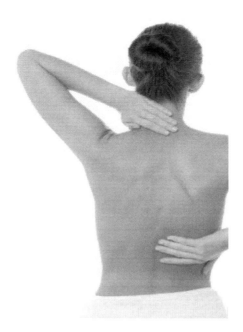

Maintains Blood Glucose and Blood Pressure

Almond oil also helps in keeping the blood pressure under control and blood glucose within normal limits.

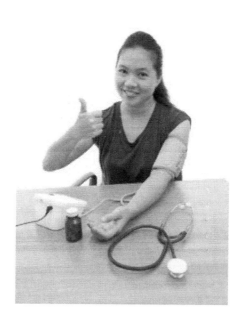

Immunity Booster

Almond oil is great for your immune system. Since it contains loads of vitamins and minerals, when taken daily it is capable of strengthening your immune system.

Vitamins and Minerals Source

Almond oil is a rich source of vitamins and minerals. It contains high amounts of calcium, potassium, magnesium, vitamins D and E. This means that if you cook in almond oil, it can be great for general health. It can also be used for salad dressing.

Strong Bones for Children

Almond oil doesn't just have benefits for adults; it is also great for little kids. All you have to do is slightly warm up some almond oil and massage it on the baby's hair and body. You can also give them a few drops of almond oil a few times a month.

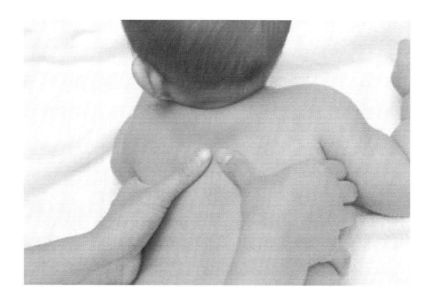

Stress Reliever

Since almond oil works as an analgesic, it helps in relieving muscular pains. If you feel stressed and there is pain in your shoulders, neck and head, then warm up almond oil and massage it to get instant relief. You will feel fresher once you have had the massage.

Aromatherapy Uses

Because of its analgesic and stress relieving properties, almond oil is used in aromatherapy and by many masseurs. Another reason for its use is that it has emollient properties, which means that is easily absorbed by the skin, leaving no oily traces. Therefore it can be mixed with other essential

oils and used for aromatherapy.

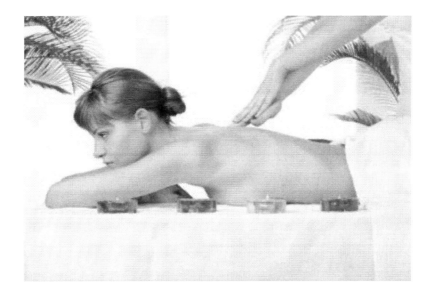

Almond Oil for Skin

Almond oil is said to be one of the most ignored beauty oils that can literally recharge your skin with continued usage. Here are some of the skin care regiments it is good for.

Soft and Smooth Skin

Is your skin becoming dull and listless? Just take some almond oil, mix it with sugar and gently rub this scrub on your face. Once you have massaged for 2 minutes, take a clean, wet cloth and wipe your face. Wash off with cold water and see the freshness. You can also use this scrub for your hands and feet.

Strong Nails

Almond oil is also an effective remedy for weak nails that refuse to grow. Simply rub some on your nails and cuticles and enjoy long and strong nails that you can paint any color you like!

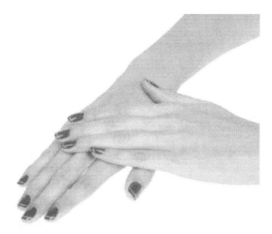

Chapped Lips

Suffering from chapped, peeling lips? Apply some almond oil. What you can do is keep a small bottle in your purse and apply whenever they feel dry. It is one of the best things that can come your way during Winter!

Enhances Eyelash Growth

Almond oil is said to work wonders for eyelashes. If you want to make them strong and long, simply mix equal amounts of almond oil and castor oil in a small bottle and apply a light coat on your lashes, just before going to bed. Brush them out and wash off in the morning. You will notice a change in just a month of daily use.

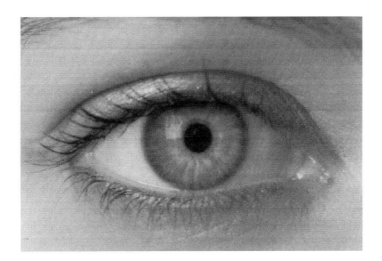

For Dark Circles

Instead of wasting money on expensive eye creams, go for something safer and more effective, almond oil! Because almond oil had anti-ageing properties, it helps clearing the dark circles, as well as the puffiness under the eyes. This way your eyes look and feel fresh. Simply take some almond oil on the tips of your fingers and gently rub it under and over your eyes. In some time you will notice that the dark circles disappear completely. But make sure you do it every day.

Wrinkle Control

As already mentioned, almond oil has anti-ageing properties which is why it can control and reduce wrinkles. You don't need to do anything except rub some almond oil on your face every night before going to bed. Make sure you run in circles and do it gently. Focus on the places where there are wrinkles.

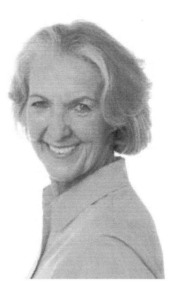

Skin Problems

If you have developed eczema or Psoriasis then almond oil can work wonders for you. The vitamins and minerals help the skin into healing quickly. Mix a few drops of chamomile essential oil and lavender essential oil in 2 tablespoons of almond oil and apply to skin 3-4 times a day. Do this for as long as it takes for the condition to heal.

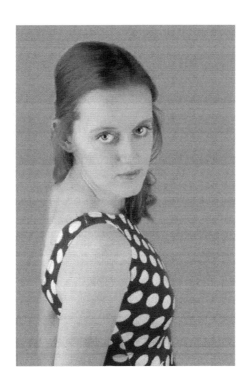

Dead Skin Remover

Suffering from a dull complexion and rough skin? Try mixing some almond oil in baking soda and rubbing it gently on your face. It is the perfect dead cell remover and works better than any commercially manufactured scrub. The almond oil gives your skin fairness and softness.

Protection from Sun

Almond oil is also believed to work well in protecting from sun. It isn't just the tan that you get saved from but also diseases like skin cancer, sunburns and even other skin conditions that occur due to the harmful effects of ultraviolet rays.

Anti-Inflammation

Redness, inflammation and soreness can all be treated with almond oil. Whether it is a minor wound, cut or abrasion on the skin or scalp, softly smooth some almond oil on it and keep doing so until completely healed.

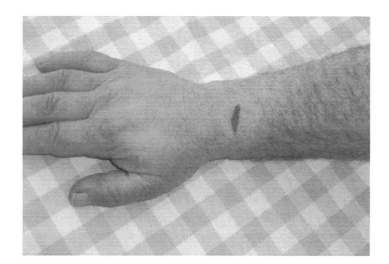

Almond Oil for Hair

Just like coconut oil and olive oil, almond oil works really well for hair. Below are all the reasons it could benefit your hair.

Long and Strong Hair

If you have short hair that refuses to grow like Rapunzel's, then almond oil may work well for you. You can either follow the same method as explained above or try something even more effective. In a glass bottle, add equal quantities of almond oil, coconut oil and 4 tablespoons of castor oil. Mix well and apply to hair. Leave in hair for at least an hour and wash off. Do this thrice a week for a minimum of 2 months.

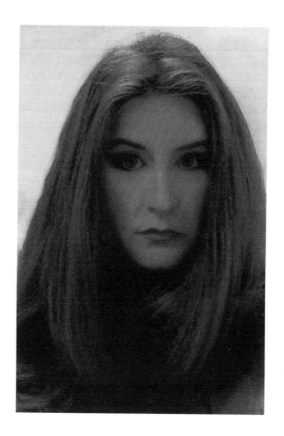

Stops Heavy Hair Falls

Have you been experiencing heavy hair fall? Then almond oil is just the cure for your falling tresses. All you need to do is warm up some oil and gently massage it into your scalp. Warm a towel and wrap it around your head in a way that all the hair is covered. Leave it on for 2 hours and then wash with warm water. Once the oil is out, wash your hair with cold water. Follow this method twice a week for 3 months. You will start seeing results within a month.

Natural Shine Enhancer

Since almond oil is a rich source of minerals and vitamins, it is a natural shine enhancer for all kinds of hair, whether dry or oily. But be sure that you apply to hair at least twice a week for lasting results.

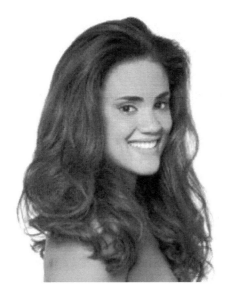

Get Rid of Dandruff

Dandruff can become a real pain during the Winter! If you too have been suffering and all else has failed, try using almond oil. Mix equal amounts of almond, coconut and olive oil and mix well before applying to the scalp. Leave it on for 2 hours and then wash thoroughly. Not only will dandruff disappear in a few days, you will also notice that your hair has become soft, shiny and strong.

Natural Leave in Conditioner

Almond oil is lightweight and gets easily absorbed in the skin and hair. So you can use it on hair for leave in conditioners. Not only will it be safer and healthier, it will also make your hair strong and long.

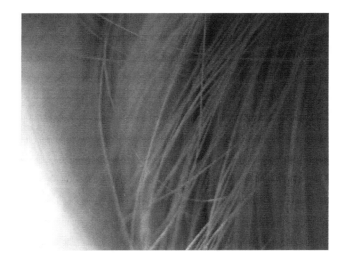

Reduces Frizz and Split Ends

Almond oil also works for split ends and frizz. Just follow the above mentioned procedures for effective results. Another thing that you can do is fill a spray bottle with water and add 3 tablespoons of almond oil and 1 tablespoon of apple cider vinegar to it. Whenever you feel that you hair is getting frizzy, spray your hair with this mixture. Don't spray too much or your hair may feel and look oily. Just a light coating will be enough.

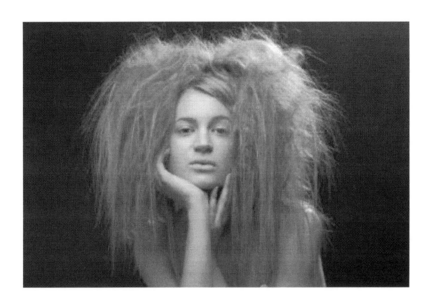

Some Easy to Use Tips and Tricks

Below are some easy homemade tips and tricks that will help you make full use of almond oil. You will have beautiful skin and hair and would wonder why you never tried these easy, natural recipes before.

Body Scrub

Have you been looking for ways to make your own body scrub that contains no harsh chemicals and is also nourishing for the skin? Try this almond oil scrub to see results that will leave you ecstatic with joy. The recipe is listed below.

Take ½ cup almond oil, 1 cup sugar, 5 capsules of vitamin E and 8-10 drops of your favorite essential oil. Take out the oil from the capsules and mix all the ingredients together. Store in an airtight jar, and use just before you take a bath. Make sure you scrub your hands, elbows, knees and feet well. Rinse off with warm water and apply moisturizer.

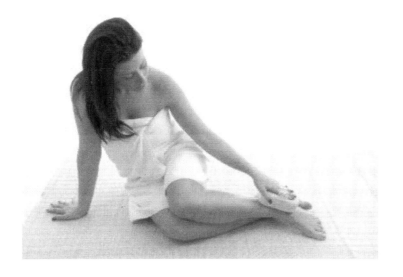

Spicy Body Oil

Want to spice up your love life? Why not make this yummy, sexy body oil and be the star of your home? It is simple, inexpensive and as harmless as can be. Here is how you can make it.

Take about ½ a cup of sweet almond oil, ¼ cup of jojoba oil, ½ cup sun seed oil, 5 drops clove essential oil, 15 drops cinnamon essential oil and 10 drops lavender essential oil. Put all these oils in a small glass bottle, shake well and use as needed. You can also add a stick of cinnamon or a few vanilla pods in the bottle to give some added spice.

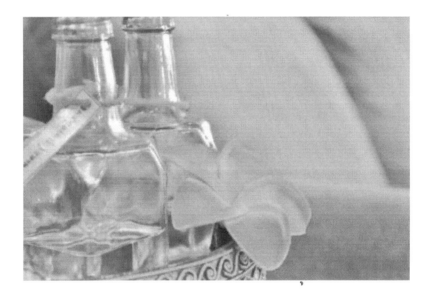

Facial Mask

The stress and pollution of your everyday routine makes the facial skin tired looking and worn. If you don't know a cheap, easy way to restore your natural beauty, here is an easy facial mask for you. This mask will also help in reducing fine lines and wrinkles.

Whisk an egg, add 1 tablespoon almond oil and 1 tablespoon coconut oil to it. Mix well and cover your face with it. Leave on for about 10 minutes and then wash off with warm water. If you don't like the smell, you can add a few drops of your favorite essential oil.

You will notice immediate results. Use the mask at least thrice a week for amazing results.

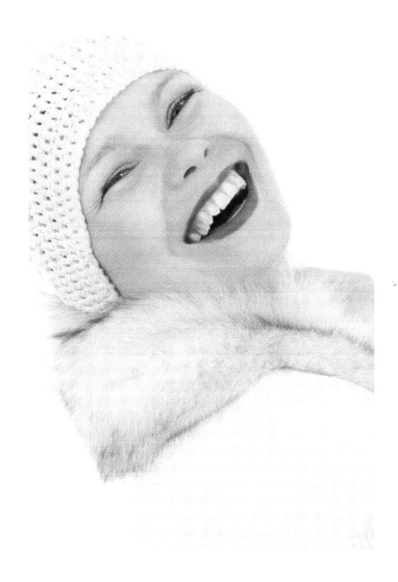

Hair Restorer

Use this hair mask for strong and beautiful hair. Don't apply the mask more than 3 times a month.

To make the mask, mix equal parts of almond oil, coconut milk and half, ripe mashed avocado.

Apply this paste to hair and cover with a shower cap. Leave on for an hour and then shampoo off.

With repeated use your dry, damaged hair will turn silky and pretty.

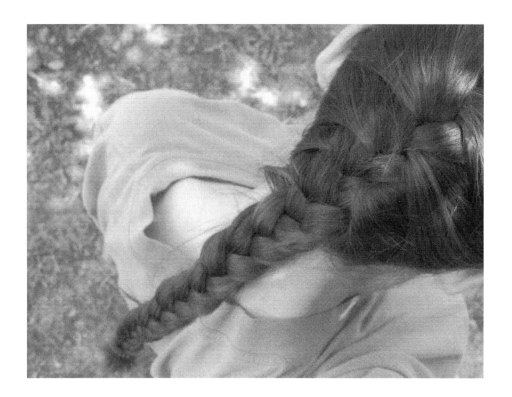

Hot Oil Treatment 1

If you don't want to spend hundreds of dollars on a hot oil treatment at a spa or a beauty parlor,

why not give yourself one right at home? It is simple, inexpensive and gives amazing results. Here

is how you can do it.

Mix 4 tablespoons almond oil, 1 tablespoon castor oil and a few drops of your favorite essential

oil or some crushed rose petals. Warm up this mixture and then massage into scalp. Cover your head with a steamed towel and leave on for an hour. Wash off with shampoo and let dry. You will

have hair that seems to shimmer like silk!

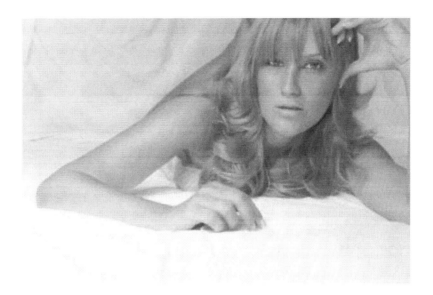

For great results, try this every week.

Hot Oil Treatment 2

You can also try this other hot oil treatment using almond oil. This too gives beautiful, shiny hair that is totally manageable.

Just take as much almond oil as you need and add a few drops of lavender essential oil to it and massage it into your scalp and hair. Then wrap a warm towel over it and leave it for an hour or two. Wash off with shampoo.

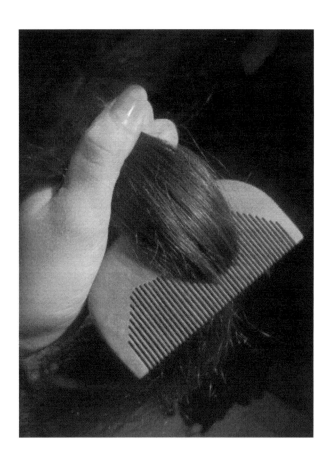

Hot Oil Treatment 2

Which Type of Almond Oil to Use

As mentioned above, almond oil is available in the form of carrier sweet almond oil and bitter essential almond oil. The latter is only used in small portions for aroma and flavor, because high dosage can be poisonous. Sweet almond oil can be used for both cooking and skin/health care.

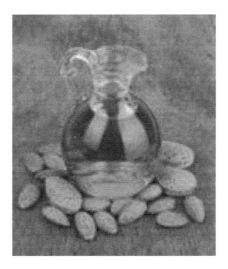

For Internal Use

There is also refined and unrefined almond oil. Experts suggest that for cooking or to be ingested orally, use refined almond oil as the unrefined version might contain some hazardous substances.

For External Use

In case of external use, it is safer to opt for refined almond oil.

Conclusion

Now that you know why apple cider vinegar, coconut oil and almond oil are so great for your

health, make sure you add them to your everyday routine. Best of luck!

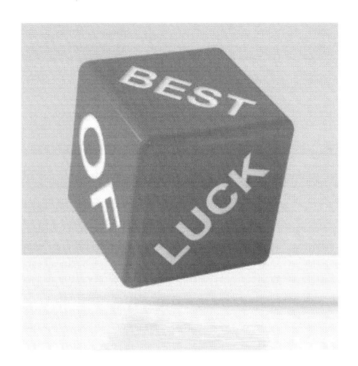

Made in the USA
Lexington, KY
14 August 2014